Sizzling Sex

Other titles of similar interest from
RANDOM HOUSE VALUE PUBLISHING, INC.

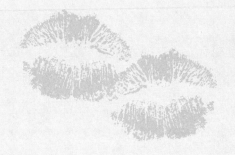

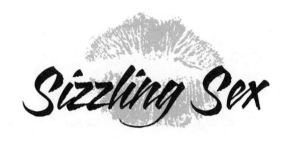

Sizzling Sex

~ 242 ~
Sure-Fire Ways
to Heat Up Your Love Life

Kirsten M. Lagatree

Gramercy Books
NEW YORK

This 2002 edition is published by Gramercy Books ™, an imprint of
Random House Value Publishing, Inc. 280 Park Avenue, New York, N.Y. 10017.

Gramercy Books™ and design are trademarks of Random House Value Publishing, Inc.

Random House
New York • Toronto • London • Sydney • Auckland
http://www.randomhouse.com/

Interior design by Lynne Amft
Printed and bound in The United States of America

Library of Congress Cataloging-in-Publication Data
Lagatree, Kirsten M.
    Sizzling sex : 242 sure-fire ways to heat up your love life / Kirsten M. Lagatree.
        p. cm.
    ISBN 0-517-21931-X
    1. Sex—Handbooks, manuals, etc. I. Title.

HQ21 .L234 2002
306.7—dc21   2001040696

9 8 7 6 5 4 3 2 1

CONTENTS

FOREWORD

If you suspect that your sex life isn't all it could be, do you know what to do about it? Are you nagged by the feeling that other people are having MORE or HOTTER sex than you are? Do you wish you knew how to make your sexual fantasies come true? If you answered yes to any of these questions, keep reading! The Tips, Tricks, Facts, and Food For Thought between these covers will heat up your life under the covers (or wherever passion strikes!).

Occasionally it helps to think of sex in terms of food. Depending on your mood — and the time available —it can be a multi-course feast, or a quick, but satisfying snack. Whatever form it takes, sex should always be served HOT!

First, let's make something clear. Heating up your sex life should bear no resemblance to warming up a can of soup or microwaving leftovers (even if that's precisely what it's been like so far). Say goodbye to sex that's as mundane as meatloaf or as predictable as Thanksgiving leftovers. With sex, food, and life itself, variety is definitely the spice!

I

Temptations and Flirtations

A great dining experience is always more enjoyable if you're hungry before you begin. Love-making is likewise more luscious when appetites have been tantalized. Here are some ideas to get those taste buds throbbing!

FACT: The most powerful sexual organ in the human body is located between the ears. Use your imagination before engaging body parts and you will have much hotter sex.

Food For Thought

"A lover without indiscretion is no lover at all."

— THOMAS HARDY, NOVELIST

TIPS
&
TRICKS | When you're in a public place, whisper that you're bra-less or let her know that there's nothing between you and your Calvins.

TIPS
&
TRICKS | 4

Suggest lewd acts in inappropriate places. It doesn't matter that you can't actually indulge yourselves there. This is definitely an occasion when "it's the thought that counts."

TIPS
&
TRICKS | 5

Propose naughty acts in places where they might indeed be carried out. Who knows what lusty feats such daring could provoke?

TIPS
&
TRICKS | 6

Here's a jumpstart for your imagination: picture the two of you coupling on a twilight beach; in the bedroom at a close friend's party (under the pile of coats, perhaps?); on a hotel balcony after sunset; under the bleachers at your home team's next ball game.

Food For Thought

*"What will not a gentle woman dare when strong affection
stirs her spirit up?"*

— Robert Southey, romantic poet

FACT — While we're on the subject of daring…visit an amusement park and go for the scream rides. A psychologist for Universal Studios Amusement Park discovered that the adrenaline rush from stomach-flipping experiences releases endorphins, which induce feelings of lust. Hold on tight….here we go!

Tips
&
Tricks | Don't assume sexy underwear is only for women and cross dressers. You'd be surprised how many guys are willing—even eager—to thrill you by tucking their stuff into a sexy satin pouch.

Tips
&
Tricks

10

Shop for sexy lingerie together. This activity will pump up both partners' pulse. The one who's trying on the dainties gets quite a rush from wearing all that sexy stuff. And the one who's watching gets a charge from imagining how delicious it will be to take those items off.

Tips
&
Tricks

11

Shop for sexy lingerie alone and surprise your partner. You can hardly go wrong picking out something the other person will be delighted with. Just knowing the article was chosen specially to tantalize him will make it very attractive indeed.

12

You don't have to answer the door in a G-string, but every now and then greet your lover dressed in something you know he thinks is sexy. When he knows that you know that he thinks it's sexy, he'll be flattered and turned on.

13

You can also send a racy signal by doing just a bit of last minute primping. The fluffed hair, fresh lipstick and splash of perfume will underscore that smoldering "come hither" look you flash him.

14

Food For Thought

"Brevity is the soul of lingerie."

— Dorothy Parker, writer

15

Buy sexier underwear for him. Anything that looks hot and is different from his usual attire. Briefer briefs or longer, tighter boxers will do the job.

16

Call or e-mail your partner during the workday with a concise, but stimulating, summary of the s-exploits you have in mind for the evening. Your preview of "coming attractions" might include anything from a candlelit bath to the debut of a naughty new video.

17

Technology doesn't have to be impersonal. Sit naked at your computer some sultry evening and send your lover messages inviting him or her to do the same. Let your fingers on the keyboard describe what your fingers (hands, arms, lips, tongue, etc.) would like to be doing if you were there in person. See how hot you can get each other as your messages delve ever deeper into your sexual fantasies.

18

Food For Thought

"I often think that a slightly exposed shoulder emerging from a long satin nightgown packed more sex than two naked bodies in bed."

— BETTE DAVIS, ACTRESS

19

FACT: To paraphrase The Jefferson Airplane, you're only as sexy as you feel. The good news is that you can be devastatingly sexy, just by building a strong sexy self image. You don't have to look like a fashion model or a movie star to drive men wild with desire. Real sexiness begins where all good sex begins, in your head!

20

TIPS & TRICKS | To gain that sexy self image, try posting positive messages to yourself in places where you'll see them often—on the refrigerator, the bathroom mirror, near your bed, and in your car. Word these notes to remind you that you are sexy and desirable *just as you are now*. Banish any notions about how you must lose ten pounds or tone up your biceps in order to feel comfortable with your body and attractive to the opposite sex. Write a note to yourself that says Sexiness is an *inside* job.

TIPS
&
TRICKS │ Spend dedicated time each week wrapped in sexy
thoughts. This daydreaming will get you in touch
with your own secret desires and give you valuable
material for some explicit and exciting pillow talk.

22

Food For Thought

"In my sex fantasy, nobody ever loves me for my mind."

— NORA EPHRON, AUTHOR AND SCREENWRITER

23

TIPS
&
TRICKS │ When she's on a business trip, tease her over the
telephone or via e-mail (if it's private!) with promises
of pleasure sessions when she gets home. Purchase a
special accessory such as massage oil or new underwear for this highly anticipated occasion.

24

While straightening his tie, picking a bit of lint from his jacket, or otherwise sprucing up your man for an important occasion, find a stray thread on his inner thigh, roll that lint brush over an erogenous zone, or give a gentle caress and pat to the seat of his pants.

25

When you're apart, do something especially romantic like writing a note featuring the words to a sexy old love song. Try quoting something classic like this ultra romantic song by George Gershwin....

"Embrace me, my sweet embraceable you
Embrace me, you irreplaceable you
Just one look at you
My heart grew tipsy in me
You and you alone
Bring out the Gypsy
in me I love all the many charms about you
Above all, I want my arms about you
Don't be a naughty baby
Come to poppa, come to poppa do
My sweet embraceable you."

26

Food For Thought

"A love song is just a caress set to music."

—SIGMUND ROMBERG, COMPOSER

27

Drop by the office when he's working late or on the weekend and seduce him on the conference table. (He'll never be bored at a board meeting again!)

28

Call him at work and read a brief passage from an erotic novel. You can choose from the classics, such as *Lady Chatterly's Lover* by D. H. Lawrence, or a bit of Victorian erotica like *Fanny Hill, Memoirs of a Woman of Pleasure*. Then again, you may want to be less literary and a little more down and dirty. It's up to you!

29

Get in the habit of being intimate with your partner in small, private ways. Call her a pet name while you're shopping for groceries; touch his arm and whisper an endearment at a party; make a reference to your most recent sexual encounter and let her know it's still on your mind. These gestures pave the way to greater sexual intimacy the next time you two are alone.

30

Men love to be told when you're in the mood. Find ways to let him know in your own private language. Your signal could be a sultry side glance, a penetrating gaze, or something as simple and quick as a wink. Depending on your personal style and your man's unique inclinations, a soft purr or an Eartha Kitt growl could also do the trick.

TIPS
&
TRICKS | Chances are your man has a secret fantasy about what he'd like to see you dressed up in. Sometime when you're together watching a movie, or a risqué ad on TV, tease him by offering to wear something similar. When you receive a positive response, file it away in your memory. Then make his jaw drop some evening when his fantasy appears at the bedroom door.

32

Food For Thought

"Modesty is a Virtue, Bashfulness is a Vice."

— BENJAMIN FRANKLIN, *POOR RICHARD'S ALMANAC*

33

TIPS
&
Tricks | When was the last time you grabbed a quickie in the car? Probably not since you've had the privacy of your own home. Try seducing your partner in the car sometime. Savor the sense of urgency, the furtive feeling that comes from this naughty change of venue.

34

Food For Thought

*"It was lovemaking, Doctor, even though it was nasty.
Maybe especially because it was nasty. Love is smutty
business, you know."*

— TOM ROBBINS, *EVEN COWGIRLS GET THE BLUES*

TIPS
&
TRICKS

35

Cuddle up together with a sexy and romantic movie.
Try *The Thomas Crown Affair* (the one with Pierce
Brosnan and Rene Russo) which has a very hot love
scene on a staircase (see "The Big Oh" for sugges-
tions on how to create your own sizzling staircase
scene). *Dirty Dancing* can be inspirational, as can
Ghost (although it might leave you a bit weepy). You
may have an easier time corralling your guy for
romantic movie night if you feature something with
a dash of macho, such as *Top Gun* or *Braveheart*.
Both also deliver in the sex and romance department
very well.

II

Kisses as Art

I n old fashioned love stories, the moment when boy
finally kisses girl represents the climax of all that has
gone before. But when real-life lovers kiss, it's usually
the prelude to the *truly* romantic part of the story, pas-
sionate lovemaking. Using the tips and tricks below will
give your kisses the tingle of old-fashioned romance
combined with shivers of modern day passion!

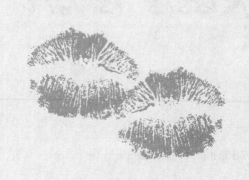

36

FACT: Kissing is important. How important? The lips have more sensitive nerve endings than any body part other than the clitoris (which has eight thousand, in case you were wondering). For most women, kissing is the most important—and most frequently under-played—element of foreplay.

37

Food For Thought

"Kisses may not spread germs, but they certainly lower resistance."

— LOUISE ERICKSON, *READER'S DIGEST*

38

TIPS
&
TRICKS

It's no coincidence that paintings of smooching lovers hang in some of the world's great museums. Kissing is an art—work on your technique until you become the Picasso of Pucker!

39

Be tender with your kisses. Intimate kissing can be the prelude to blissful sex if you approach it sensitively.

40

Be as provocative as possible, but begin slowly and allow passion to build gradually. It's just like The Supremes' mom always used to say…"you can't hurry love, no you can't hurry love…!"

41

Use your kisses to communicate, as well as stimulate, desire. Letting the other person feel your own mounting passion is a big part of the thrill in a Major Kiss.

42

Food For Thought

"Her lips suck forth my soul."

— Christopher Marlowe, *Dr. Faustus*

43

Tips & Tricks | To ensure maximum possible kissing rapture, sit (or stand) very close, taking care not to pin anyone's arms. Arms must be free to roam at will, going wherever whim or passion dictates in any given moment.

44

Tips & Tricks | Keep in mind that a deeply satisfying kiss requires more than just the lip lock. Caress your lover's face, hair, arms, chest, back, thighs—you get the idea.

45

Don't forget those tiny, out of the way places.
Kiss your lover's eye corners, ear lobes, neck, wrists,
and other delicate parts.

46

For a spine tingling thrill, gently whirl your
fingers around the ridges and hollows of your
partner's ear. Breathe gently into an ear while deftly
lapping at those inner hollows.

47

A truly cosmic kissing session includes soft,
moist and gentle nuzzling. Nudge your nose into as
many sensitive spots as possible.

48

Giving an open-mouthed neck kiss while sucking, licking, and nibbling that tender area can drive your lover wild. Of course, it can also drive a ticklish person wild with squirming and giggling. Be sure you know which reaction you're provoking!

49

For a richly provocative kiss, nibble a top or bottom lip and suck delicately on upper and lower lips.

50

Practice a bit of Oriental wisdom by having him lick your upper lip. According to some Asian philosophies, this spot corresponds to your clitoris; giving it special attention rushes an urgent message to Sex Central.

51

FACT: The area above the front teeth is surprisingly rich in sensitive nerve endings. Use your tongue to probe behind your lover's upper lip.

52

Tips
&
Tricks

Too much tongue too soon can be a real turn off. Take your cues from your lover's breathing. Don't move to the next stage of the kiss until you've gauged your partner's readiness.

53

Tips
&
Tricks

Explore the innermost reaches of his mouth with your tongue. Can you touch the soft tissue behind his palette? The roof of his mouth is very sensitive with many highly attuned nerve endings.

54

Start this oral discovery expedition by using your tongue to circle his lips, then lick beneath and behind them. Some men have particularly sensitive lower lips. You can playfully bite and nibble.

55

As passion increases, allow your kisses to stray further from the lips, but don't forget to return to home plate every now and then.

56

When the atmosphere has warmed sufficiently, begin to suck your partner's tongue. This move demonstrates true intimacy and a willingness to "meld" with your lover. It's also highly suggestive of you-know-what.

57

Food For Thought

"Red hair she had and golden skin,
Her sulky lips were shaped for sin."

— SIR JOHN BETJEMAN, 20TH CENTURY BRITISH POET

III

Sense-sational Foreplay

Foreplay is to sex what stretching is to exercise. Well, sort of. At the very least, foreplay limbers up the players for the action to come and ultimately makes lovemaking more satisfying for both partners. Although foreplay is essential to high quality sex, even women sometimes try to take shortcuts because they're "stuck" for creative foreplay ideas. With the tips below, you'll never be at a loss again.

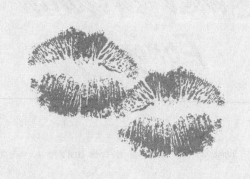

58

FACT: Set your stopwatch! A Kinsey report found that nearly 95 percent of women whose lovers spent more than 20 minutes on foreplay reached orgasm.

59

Food For Thought

"It's not the men in your life. It's the life in your men."

— MAE WEST, ACTRESS

60

TIPS **&** TRICKS

Observing The Golden Rule will add a knowing touch to your foreplay. Chances are that your lover is unconsciously doing unto you things he would love to have done to him. For example, if he twiddles your nipples, that's a pretty good indication that his nipples are one of his hot erogenous zones. Don't take this too literally; don't begin mirroring his moves immediately. Just file a few ideas away to try out the next time.

61

As you fantasize about foreplay, think about the five senses. You don't have to be systematic about it, just give a little thought to the ways you would like to tantalize each of your lover's senses during love-making — and how you would enjoy being tantalized. You will each enjoy a deeper, wider and wilder sexual experience when you practice this.

62

FACT: In a Loyola University study both men and women found the same three colors to be erotic: red-orange, dark blue, and violet. Both sexes also found gray to be, well, gray.

63

Use erotic colors to transform your bedroom into a den of provocation and pleasure. But go easy. If you don't look your best in the number one hot and sexy shade, don't swath yourself or the room in it.

64

Purchase draperies, sheets, candles, lampshades, and other accessories in a variety of coordinating erotic colors.

65

FACT: Although men tend to be more visual than women where sexual arousal is concerned, women, apparently have begun to catch up. In several surveys, both sexes reported being turned on by watching their lovers undress. The more provocatively done, of course, the better!

66

Take advantage of this opportunity for eroticism and use a bit of finesse when undressing. You don't have to be Brigitte Bardot to do the job with a certain *je ne sais quoi*. Take your time and savor the reaction your seductive strip tease is producing.

T IPS

&

T RICKS

67

Treat your partner to an eye-popping posterior view. Both men and women should find occasions to bend over naked every now and then. Displaying the genitals in such an unexpected way — with just a hint of the submissive to it—will call forth the animal instinct in even the most distracted spouse.

T IPS

&

T RICKS

68

Since men do, in fact, respond very well to visual stimuli, interested women should dress accordingly — and provocatively. But remember, what he doesn't see can be sexier than what he does. No need to get yourself up in a way that would make Britney Spears blush. Less isn't *always* more.

69

Food For Thought

"No woman so naked as one you can see to be naked underneath her clothes."

—M ICHAEL F RAYN, PLAYWRIGHT

70

Find out what turns your man on, then wear it when you have a rendezvous. His ego won't be the only thing that swells when he sees that you've dressed just to please him.

71

If your man is one of the many who ogles women in sheer blouses, give him special opportunities to ogle *you*. Invite him to lunch sometime and wear your sheer blouse under a suit jacket. Flash him a glimpse every now and then during your special meal. Dessert will be sweet and gooey.

72

Make sure he can watch while you pleasure him with your mouth. Not only does he spin into orbit from the physical sensations, he gets a great view looking down at earth.

Tips
&
Tricks | Mirrors add dimension to foreplay and intercourse. Watching yourselves in the mirror while making love adds a slightly voyeuristic element and can intensify the sheer pleasure of the act, which takes on an exciting theatrical aspect.

74

FACT: The chief distraction for women during sex is preoccupation with how they look. When a woman is wondering if her thighs are too big or if her tummy is jiggling, she isn't enjoying lovemaking and is unlikely to have an orgasm.

75

Food For Thought

"The average man is more interested in a woman who is interested in him than he is in a woman with beautiful legs."

—MARLENE DIETRICH, ACTRESS

76

A woman should purchase lingerie that makes her feel sexy, desirable, and comfortable. There's no need to stuff yourself into a teddy if you don't like the way it looks or feels. The choices are vast enough so every woman can be a babe in bed.

77

Keep the lighting indirect. Overhead bulbs are harsh and can be depressing and unromantic as well as unflattering.

78

Candlelight creates a romantic atmosphere *and* casts a flattering glow over a less than perfect body. Use sturdy, long burning drip-less candles. Just one or two flickering nearby will turn the two of you into the stars of your own steamy foreign flick.

79

Food For Thought

"Sex appeal is fifty percent what you've got and fifty percent what people think you've got."

—SOPHIA LOREN, ACTRESS

TIPS
&
TRICKS

80

To create a similar visual effect without candles, replace a standard light bulb with a red one. You'll feel positively wicked in your homemade red light district.

TIPS
&
TRICKS

81

Sure it creates a mysterious flickering light, but under no circumstances should you leave the *television* on! The only exception to this rule is if you're both overcome by passion while watching an erotic video and the urgency of the moment prevents you from reaching for the remote.

82

Nobody ever said you have to take all your clothes off to have sex. In fact, some of the sexiest sex is to be had while lingerie or clothing is pushed out of the way of throbbing body parts.

83

FACT: Oh baby! Hearing appreciative sounds during sex is a big turn on for both men and women. And take note, probably the only time a guy wants you to tell him what to do is during sex. So take advantage of it. (Oh yeah....There! There! Faster!)

TIPS
&
TRICKS

84

Learn to enjoy talking dirty. Let yourself get carried away in bed using all those words that aren't acceptable in polite conversation. This is not the time for biology book words like "vagina" and "penis."

Tips & Tricks

85

A simple way to practice your bed patter is to comment on how you're feeling at various high points. Or better yet, comment on how good he's making you feel. For example, "When you touch me like that, it drives me wild," or, "It feels incredible to have you inside me." Choose your moments based on what you're really feeling and never fake it. If you feel phony, you'll sound that way—a definite mood killer.

Tips & Tricks

86

Play romantic music to enhance the ambiance of your romancing. Be sure to consider the atmosphere you want to establish when you're selecting tunes. Music you both loved at a rock concert may not convey quite the right mood for making love.

87

Food For Thought

"My music isn't supposed to make you wanna riot! My music is supposed to make you wanna fuck!"

— JANIS JOPLIN, SINGER

88

FACT: *Take Five*, anyone? Jazz listeners have the most sex, according to the folks at the National Opinion Research Center in Chicago. Dave Brubeck is only one sexy choice among many, of course.

TIPS
&
TRICKS

89

Romantic or sexy music is in the ear of the beholder. Don't ask him to name the song from your first date, just play it. It will register, particularly if you treat him the way you did that day.

90

FACT: Chocolate stimulates the production of dopamine in the brain and increases a woman's sex drive.

91

Tips
&
Tricks | Duh! Bring her candy.

92

Tips
&
Tricks | Hold tiny bites of her favorite candy between your teeth and coax her to nibble the sweets from your lips.

93

Tips
&
Tricks | If she's a real chocoholic—or if he is—by all means purchase chocolate body paint.

TIPS
&
TRICKS | **94**

You needn't stop at chocolate, of course, and you don't even need to shop for body paint. Depending on personal taste, you can certainly experiment with luscious lickables from whipped cream to peanut butter.

TIPS
&
Tricks | **95**

Hint: Choose smooth rather than hairy places to apply body edibles. Even in the throws of passion, you may find that hair and food are not the most pleasant combination.

TIPS
&
TRICKS | **96**

If you want to taste good without the toppings, avoid spicy foods, red meat, alcohol, and garlic for several hours before you plan to swap bodily fluids. Aside from what they may do to your breath, these foods can give your secretions a bitter tang.

97

Food For Thought

"Pizza is a lot like sex. When it's good, it's really good.
When it's bad, it's still pretty good."

— ANONYMOUS

98

FACT: The folks who devote time to discovering such things at The Smell and Taste Treatment and Research Foundation in Chicago, claim that certain aromas and tastes can exert a powerful influence on the kind of love you'll make.

TIPS
&
TRICKS

99

Women, dab lavender oil on your neck and hair to turn your man into a snorting, pawing stallion.

100

FACT: To make that pants pony prance, feed a man oranges. They boost blood flow to the penis by 20 percent.

101

Feast on strawberries and cream in bed. The combination makes for an erotic picnic and the strawberries increase ultimate satisfaction for both sexes.

102

The aroma of allspice, cinnamon, and nutmeg will make you hungry for more sex (and possibly apple pie).

103

Begin your time together with a scented bath. Don't forget the flower petals.

TIPS & TRICKS | 104

Anyone who's ever seen the movie *Tom Jones* (and if you haven't, add it to your list for private movie night) knows just how lusty enjoying a meal together can be. Women, don't make the mistake of thinking that eating like a bird will make you seem more feminine and alluring. Remember that indulging appetites fully is what sex and sexiness is all about.

TIPS & TRICKS | 105

If you choose scented candles for your boudoir, find out whether your partner has allergies that could lead to more nose-blowing than mind-blowing. Also, make sure the fragrance is not so strong that it detracts from the sexy natural aromas of your bodies.

106

Even if your idea of hot sex is hordes of hunky
firemen charging your bedroom with hoses
extended, never leave a burning candle alone. And
always place candles on a fireproof surface such as
tiles or saucers.

107

Never underestimate the power of your natural
body scent! Provided you are fresh and clean, the
smells that waft from your body during lovemaking
are among nature's most potent aphrodisiacs.

108

Create tactile anticipation. Begin your caresses
on the less sensitive parts of your lover's body such as
the shoulders, arms, and hips, then move gradually
to more delicate and tender areas such as the neck,
temples, inner arms, inner thighs, etc.

109

Try a body to body rubdown. Have one partner (preferably the man) lie face down on any comfortable surface. Rub your face against his neck, your breasts against his back, and begin moving down, using the length of your body to rub his. Give plenty of time to rubbing breasts against buttocks.

110

To set the mood when you're relaxing together, ever so lightly scratch her back, shoulders, arms, legs, buttocks…begin whispering what you plan to do a little later.

111

The instep and interior part of the ankle are very susceptible to soft caresses, nibbles, and tongue kisses.

IV

Sexcessories

For some lovers, using accessories is the most natural thing in the world. For others, no matter how curious or interested they may be, the notion of sex toys seems somewhere just to the north of bestiality. Relax, incorporating sex toys into lovemaking may not be for everyone, but it's certainly as "normal" as good old American rhubarb pie!

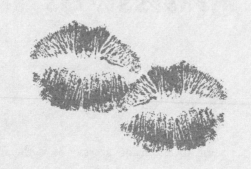

112

FACT: A recent survey found that the typical user of sex toys is married, monogamous, and college educated. The most popular sex toys are vibrators and dildos, but there's an entire world of novelty items out there just waiting to be explored by the curious and adventuresome.

113

TIPS
&
TRICKS
If you think you might be interested in experimenting with sex toys, spend some time browsing sex shops or specialty Web sites. Don't feel pressured into buying right away; there are dozens and dozens of items out there, take your time doing the research.

114

TIPS
&
TRICKS
Surf some sex Web sites with your partner. Turn this research project into a sexual bonding (not bondage) experience for the two of you. Use the occasion to discuss not just the sex aids themselves, but your feelings about using them.

115

Food For Thought

"There are a number of mechanical devices which increase sexual arousal, particularly in women. Chief among these is the Mercedes-Benz 380SL convertible."

— P.J. O'ROURKE, WRITER

TIPS
&
TRICKS

116

Don't get uptight about using—or not using— sex toys. Some couples experiment with them a few times and decide they prefer sex the old fashioned way—no technology or novelty items involved. Other couples use them every now and then for novelty and to keep their lovemaking fresh. Either way is fine, as long as both you and your partner are happy with your choice.

TIPS
&
TRICKS

117

Keep in mind that using sex toys is normal and not using sex aids is also normal. It is purely a matter of individual preference.

118

Whatever you decide, you will gain intimacy
from talking about the issue. It can be an excellent
way of exploring your feelings together and learning
more about yourselves and each other.

119

The primary advantage of any sexual aid is to race
your human engine by adding novelty to the routine.

120

FACT: The first vibrators became available in the late 1800's.
But they were available only to doctors to dole out as
needed to female patients suffering from anxiety,
irritability, "pelvic heaviness" and "excessive" vaginal
lubrication. In our less restrained modern parlance,
that would be horniness. During World War I, ads
began appearing in magazines offering electric
vibrators to women as a home remedy for hysteria,
which was understood to be genitally induced.

121

A "sex toy" can be anything from an ice cube to a silk scarf. Use that racy imagination of yours to come up with ideas.

122

Sometimes the most humble home furniture can become a truly magnificent accessory to sex. For example, a kitchen stool can be turned into a special seat for pleasure. The woman perches on the edge and arches back, leaning her elbows on the stool, and exposing a luscious mid-morning snack to her kneeling partner.

123

For the slightly more adventurous, the same stool can provide the perfect prop for a woman leaning over face down. In this position her vulva should be just the right height for a spectacular sensation with the right combination of lover's lips, fingers, and tongue.

124

For "soft bondage" sex, tie your partner's hands loosely with scarves, wide satin ribbon, or any silky material. When hands are restrained, the "victim" has a more intense physical experience. Unable to initiate pleasure, he or she can focus only on receiving it.

125

Blindfold one partner during lovemaking. Deprived of sight, and the ability to watch what's going on, the body's other senses kick into high gear to compensate, intensifying other physical sensations. A silky scarf also works well for this because the feel of the material adds to the sensual experience.

126

Food For Thought

"Sticks and stones may break my bones. But whips and chains excite me."

—ANONYMOUS

127

FACT: Steamy movies are not just for the stained raincoat crowd anymore. Just as sex toys have gone mainstream, erotic videos are also finding a wider audience. In fact, a study by The Archives of Sexual Behavior in Britain found that women get just as big a charge out of watching erotica as men do.

128

Until fairly recently, adult films were produced by men for men. Your choices are wider and more appealing now. Look for adult movie companies that specialize in films produced for women and couples. (e.g., Femme Productions in New York City)

129

Purchase massage oils in an assortment of aromas (or flavors) that you both enjoy. Sensual massage will become a more frequent part of foreplay when you're stocked up and ready to roll ahead of time.

130

A full-body massage can be an exquisite entry to foreplay, or it can be an end in itself. Have your lover lie down on a bed or soft, thick carpet protected with sheets or towels. The massage will be more enjoyable for both of you if your partner is naked and freshly showered. Begin at the shoulders and neck, kneading firmly but gently to ease away the stress that collects in these areas. Next, work your way down the arms to press, knead and squeeze the hands, palms and fingertips. Continue massaging the entire body, using your whole hand and your outstretched fingers and touching every part of your partner's body as rhythmically and lovingly as possible. Don't break the spell with quick, jerky or rough hand movements. You may, of course, embroider on this basic formula to kick the action up a notch into foreplay (tease nipples, suck fingers or toes after massaging them, run fingertips lightly over inner thigh and groin areas, etc.). Or, you may prefer to focus solely on the relaxation and delicious languor you can create for your lover. Either way, this experience will provide pleasure for you both and enhance the closeness between you.

131

Buy a good sexual lubricant and keep it within easy reach. Even if you don't think you particularly need one, you'll enjoy the new dimension it adds to foreplay and mutual fondling.

132

A quality lubricant is also indispensable to the pleasure of *both* partners in prolonged or frequent intercourse. But use caution not to over-lubricate, lest you lose all friction.

V

Sexercise

As we've pointed out, you don't need the body of an athlete or super model to enjoy a sublime sexual relationship with your partner. "Come as you are" (as it were) should definitely be the first rule of play. That said, it never hurts to make sure all your important equipment is in the best possible working order. The coyly named "sexercises" suggested here will add to your ultimate pleasure and probably won't be too burdensome a way to spend your spare moments.

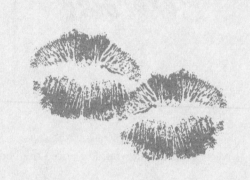

133

FACT: Studies show that 30 minutes of aerobic exercise three times a week is very good for your sex life. It raises testosterone levels, thus boosting libido; increases blood flow, which makes genital tissue more responsive to pleasure; and improves cardiovascular endurance, which allows you to enjoy yourself much longer.

TIPS
&
TRICKS

134

Here's the beauty part: Sex itself is great exercise. But you can see the dilemma immediately if you don't get enough exercise *outside* the bedroom, you may not find yourself *in* the bedroom as often. So don't think of exercise as work, think of it as fore-play.

135

FACT: While we're on the subject of good health and great sex, here's another excellent reason to quit smoking cigarettes. In addition to rotting your lungs, the nasty weed also constricts blood flow to those vital organs, the vagina and penis. Studies also show that nicotine depresses testosterone levels, which lowers the sex drive in both men and women.

136

TIPS & TRICKS

Learn to love living lean. The lower your body fat, the higher your testosterone level. As we know, the higher your testosterone level, the higher your sex drive. Let the gravy boat pass you by and catch the Love Boat instead.

137

Try this exercise—guys will love it and women will reap the rewards. The woman kisses and caresses her partner while he lies still without responding. That's it—that's the exercise! But here's the catch: if a man has trouble enjoying these caresses for at least 20 minutes, chances are he's a bit hasty in the foreplay department. Repeat this drill until he accomplishes the 20-minute minimum. Lucky him.

138

FACT: Kegel exercises for women strengthen the muscle that contracts when you have an orgasm—and when that muscle is stronger, so are your orgasms. Do Kegel exercises to tone up your pleasure zone.

Tips
&
Tricks

139

Here's how simple a Kegel is: Contract and relax the muscle that allows you to control your flow of urine. You are flexing your pubococcygeal, or PCP muscle. Flex it a few dozen times a day, and within weeks you will notice a difference in the duration and intensity of your climaxes.

Tips
&
Tricks

140

If you have trouble locating the right muscle, zero in on it by practicing while peeing.

Tips
&
Tricks

141

Do your Kegels while you're stuck in traffic, sipping your morning coffee, talking on the telephone, applying makeup, enduring a dull meeting, reading this book, anywhere, anytime…. No one will have a clue what you're up to!

142

Tips & Tricks

Here's another nifty thing to do with that buff PCP muscle. Squeeze and release it while your is partner is thrusting inside you and thrill him with something unexpected. Ask him to tell you how and when he likes it best.

143

FACT: Don't beg off sex because of a headache, try begging for it instead. The female orgasm, as it happens, releases endorphins and is a powerful painkiller.

VI

Playing Doctor
by Yourself

You'd be surprised how many women still don't think they should touch themselves "down there." And heck, if they won't do it, how are they ever going to feel comfortable letting anyone else do it? Much less make sure they do it right? Read on...

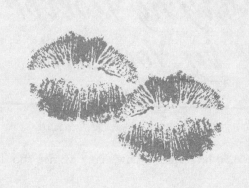

144

FACT: The clitoris is made of erectile tissue, just like the penis. Despite its dainty size (it averages 16 millimeters, a little over half an inch), the clitoris has more nerve endings and is more sensitive to direct touch than the penis.

145

TIPS
&
TRICKS | Here's the most important thing to understand about the clitoris: its only function is to give pleasure to a woman. How's that for a *vital* organ?

146

Food For Thought

"Know thyself."

— PLUTARCH, GREEK PHILOSOPHER

147

Plutarch probably wasn't talking to women about orgasms when he coined that phrase, but it's good advice all the same. Women who know their bodies —who know where, how, and when they want to be touched—will have orgasms more easily and more often than women who don't.

148

Food For Thought

"Recently, when I am alone I try to talk myself out of masturbation. I ask myself why can't I just be friends with myself."

— RICHARD LEWIS, COMEDIAN

149

Don't worry about going blind or growing hair on your palms. The way you'll get frequent orgasms is the same way you'll get to Carnegie Hall. Practice! Practice! Practice!

150

Before you get started, take time to put yourself in the mood. As part of your "practice," luxuriate in a fragrant bath, read an erotic story, or enjoy any activity that awakens your sensual nature.

151

Approach your clitoris with gentle and even indirect touches. Start with panties on and stroke it lightly through the fabric with your fingernail.

152

Using your fingers or a vibrator, experiment with different touches, intensities, and speeds on every part of your vaginal area.

153

Use lubrication at first until your body begins to respond by pumping out some of its own.

154

Food For Thought

"A girl with brains ought to do something better with them than think."

— Anita Loos, author, *Gentlemen Prefer Blondes*

155

Try this yourself and then teach your man the three-fingered technique: use your index, middle and ring finger together to massage your clitoris. This configuration is just right for touching every sensitive nerve ending at once.

156

By all means, branch out. Don't limit your explorations to the clitoris. Delve into all the voluptuous folds and valleys that make up your vulva: the large and small lips, known technically as the labia majora and minora; your clitoral hood (just what it sounds like); and the opening, or vestibule of your vagina. Notice what each feels like before and after arousal.

157

FACT: Yes, Virginia, there is a G-Spot and every woman has one. It's a bump an inch or so up your vaginal wall on the front (belly) side. When you press this spot, you may first feel the urge to urinate—the G-Spot is actually the urethral sponge.

TIPS & TRICKS

158

Despite its renown as a magic sexual gizmo, the G-Spot is not *the* spot for every woman. So don't be discouraged if yours doesn't respond the way some articles and sex manuals promise it will. But it's definitely worth checking yours out.

TIPS & TRICKS

159

For best results, give your G-Spot a test run right after you've emptied your bladder and when you're already slightly aroused. Lie on your back and slip your index finger into your vagina until you feel a bump. Using a "come here" motion, stimulate the spot gently. Be patient, wait for sensations to materialize, and don't expect an immediate or dramatic reaction. Try this a few times until you've become acquainted with your little friend, G.

160

FACT: Good news for guys: you have G-spots, too. The bad news, however: it's that condom-sized gland you hoped you'd never have to think much about. Yes, fellas, your G-spot is your P-spot—P as in prostate. It can be accessed via your perineum—the patch of skin half-way between the base of the scrotum and the anus.

161

TIPS
&
Tricks

Here's the "Up The Down Staircase" method of accessing the male G-spot. Insert a well-lubricated finger gently into the rectum, and slowly move it in and out. This works best if you start when he's already aroused. Begin making come-hither motions with your finger. You are now knock-knock-knockin' on heaven's door.

162

Here's a method of reaching that G-spot without
going up the down staircase. With a lubricated hand,
stroke his penis until he's close to orgasm. With the
index finger of your other hand, press and caress his
perineum firmly enough to stimulate the prostate
gland (G-spot) nestled up inside.

163

Either of these G-spot maneuvers works
extremely well when combined with oral sex.
But you've probably thought of this by now.

164

While it's vital for women to get to know their own bodies, it's also an excellent idea for them to learn a thing or two about the penis. Women shouldn't make the mistake of assuming that his throbbing tower of erectile tissue responds in any way like your dainty little mini version. The clitoris and the penis may be made of similar material, but they want very different kinds of treatment.

165

Because the clitoris contains many more nerve endings than the penis, it requires only a gentle touch, at least in the early stages of foreplay. A penis is made of sterner, somewhat less delicate stuff, and responds best to a fairly firm grip. Use about the same pressure you would in a business-like hand-shake.

166

The most sensitive area of the penis is the part that looks a little like a fireman's hat at the end of the shaft. It's known as the glans, or head. The most sensitive spot on the glans is a little seam on the underside of this tissue that connects the head to shaft. The rim around the bottom of the fireman's hat and the long ridge that runs the length of the underside of the penis are two other worthwhile destinations for your tongue, hands, and fingers.

167

FACT: There is no truth to the rumor that larger penises become huge and ultra potent instruments in the erect state, dwarfing and outperforming their smaller brethren. Researchers Masters and Johnson actually conducted size experiments in their laboratory and discovered that relatively smaller flaccid penises (3 to $3\frac{1}{2}$ inches long) roughly doubled in size when erect. But larger organs (measuring approximately 4 to $4\frac{3}{4}$ inches) gained only an average of $2\frac{3}{4}$ to 3 inches when fully expanded. In any case, as most women will tell you, the question is moot since the primary action for her arousal is the clitoral caress, not the piston pump.

168

For both men and women, the most important piece of sexual advice is to let your partner know what you like in bed. If you're not used to doing this (and an astonishing number of adults are not), this can be tough, even if you've been together for a while. But if you choose your moments prudently, you'll both be glad you did.

169

If you feel intimidated by talking about what you like to have done to your body, look at it this way: wouldn't you want to know how to please your partner? Wouldn't you feel delighted by the trust your partner demonstrated in you? Wouldn't you also feel a sexual thrill knowing you had the power to drive him or her wild in bed? Withholding information doesn't do either of you any good and it may even erode the relationship down the road.

170

Whenever you can do it, your best bet is to make your preferences known in the heat of the moment. A timely cue for an attentive partner can be as simple as, "Oh, yes…there! Like that!" or "Mmmmmm… a little to the right, " "faster, harder, softer," and so on.

171

You have nothing to gain and much to lose by keeping your desires a secret. Face it, since men and women are wired so deliciously differently, and neither sex possesses mind reading ability, it is impossible to guess what the other person is feeling (or not feeling).

VII

The Birds, the Bees, and the S.T.D.'S

Let's face it, if you're embarrassed to bring up the subject of condoms, or are afraid your concerns about safe sex will fall on deaf ears, maybe this isn't someone you ought to be having sex with. But we're not here to lecture you (ok, just that one sentence). The purpose of this book is to help you have fun with sex. But it's sure no fun to be worried about whether you might catch something dreadful or fatal while you're swapping fluids. So swallow your embarrassment before you swallow absolutely anything else and use these tips to keep yourself and your close personal friends happy and healthy.

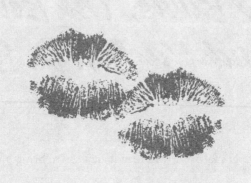

172

FACT: Eighty-three percent of heterosexual adults have
        never had a sexually transmitted disease. But don't
        let that statistic lull you into a false sense of security.
        If you do the math, you'll see that number leaves just
        under twenty percent who *have* had some form of
        STD. Even if you think you're not at risk for
        AIDS/HIV (and there's no such person, the risks are
        just higher for some than others), any time you have
        unprotected sex, you're still an excellent candidate
        for AIDS or any of the others. To refresh your mem-
        ory, those include herpes, gonorrhea, chlamydia,
        syphilis, urethritis, or pelvic inflammatory disease
        (PID). Did we mention hepatitis?

173

FACT: The only way to be absolutely sure that you are not at
        risk for contracting an STD is to remain in a monog-
        amous relationship that has lasted for at least 10
        years, or to wear a condom every time you have
        intercourse.

174

Safe sex doesn't have to be unromantic or boring, You'll get cooperation from even the most condom-phobic partner when you offer to put the penis poncho on with your mouth.

175

Hold the condom with the rolled edge facing you and place it between your lips and teeth. Now stick your tongue into the condom, pushing the tip out just past your lips. Place your condom-tipped tongue on the tip of his penis and unroll the condom over it with your lips, which are carefully covering your teeth. Be sure to leave some space at the tip for the semen. To practice this technique, pick up a banana at the produce section of your supermarket (take it home first!).

176

Remember that petroleum-based lubricants will break down the fiber in latex condoms and block their effectiveness. If you're using a condom, stay away from home products like baby oil, hand lotion, and Vaseline. You can, however, use any vegetable oil or simply purchase a water-based jelly like KY, which is easily available in the drug store.

177

The safest of all possible sexual activities are those that don't require protection. These include massage, mutual masturbation, body-to-body rubdowns, stripteases, exhibitionism, fantasy role playing, dry kissing, and anything else you can think of that doesn't involve the swapping of body fluids. Abstinence, of course, is safe. But it ain't sex, and it's not always reliable.

VIII

The Big OH!

Who knows why Nature created the orgasm? After all, lots of us would go ahead and mess around even without the big payoff, just because it's kinda fun. But then again, sex can be inconvenient and it's often messy. Sometimes you even have to go to the trouble of taking all your clothes off and putting them back on. Since you're going to all this trouble for sex, use these tips to make sure you get the big bang Nature intended.

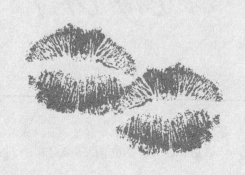

178

FACT: An orgasm a day keeps the doctor away. As if there weren't enough reasons to enjoy them! In the 1980s a study at a Detroit psychiatric clinic found that patients' overall health improved along with their sex lives as the frequency of orgasms increased.

179

Food For Thought

"The ability to make love frivolously is the chief characteristic which distinguishes human beings from beasts."

—Heywood Hale Broun, journalist and author

180

FACT: Vaginal orgasms are the exception, not the rule. Research shows that 70 percent of women experience orgasm mainly through clitoral stimulation.

181

There are ways to get that magic button pushed during intercourse. With your man on top and inside, have him shift slightly higher up your torso. This puts his penis at a steeper angle so it rubs against your clitoral hood.

182

Yet another clever clit caressing trick is an ancient Arabian position known as *dok el arz* (pounding the spot). The man sits with his legs stretched out in front; the woman sits astride his thighs, crosses her legs behind his back, and guides his penis inside. She wraps her arms around his neck while he places his arms around her waist so he can help her pump up and down on him.

183

Drink a can of Coke about 10 minutes before making love. The caffeine and the sugar will give your orgasm a special rush. Things go (and come) better with coke!

184

Women can skip the soft drink and still have a major blast-off by concentrating on breathing. Take slow, regular breaths as your arousal builds. When you feel orgasm approaching, inhale deeply a few times and consciously relax the muscles in your pelvic region.

185

Conversely, a woman close to orgasm who feels the goal slip-sliding away can often hurtle herself across the finish line by tensing her arms, legs, and stomach.

186

If your man is about to gallop through the finish line while you are trotting at a more leisurely pace, there is a way to reign him in very pleasantly. As his climax nears, encircle his scrotum with your thumb and fingers and tug—very gently — pulling down lightly on his scrotum. Once you master this technique, you'll provide ecstasy for him and catch up time for you.

187

Just for fun, arouse your man's penis without touching it. You can do this any number of ways, but suggestive sucking on other digits is a great way to start. Flick your tongue in and out of his ears, kiss and caress the nape of his neck, then move lower to lick and suck his nipples, chest and stomach. Pay special attention to his bottom, kissing, nibbling and licking his buns and darting your tongue between and just beneath his cheeks. Nuzzle his testicles, fondle and suck his scrotum while fingering his perineum (that spot between scrotum and anus). He should be hard as a rock and begging for mercy by this time.

188

Try this version of the "Adam and Eve." The man should stand up with feet planted firmly about shoulder width apart. The woman crouches low into a snake position and slithers up between his calves and through his thighs. She should press her breasts as sensually as possible against his inner thighs, scrotum, and belly. She continues to wrap herself slowly around his trunk from behind, and takes her time before she moves around to stand face to face.

189

With both lovers nude, the woman stands facing the man, her bare feet on top of his, her breasts pressed firmly against his chest, and holding on to him very tight. His hard penis then slides between her legs. Be sure there's enough lubrication for this joy ride. Now, she should ask him to walk around the room, the yard, the block with her.

190

For an orgasmic workout, have him lie on a weight bench as if he were going to do his bench press. Now that he's planted on a good foundation, with his hips slightly elevated, he's in just the right position for you to saddle up. Unlike equestrians, you may indeed sit on the saddle horn. Try various angles with different speeds. You might even want to mount up riding backwards for a special thrill.

191

Hammocks provide for natural swing on those hot sultry days when we want a minimum of movement but maximum sensation. A light skimpy sundress for her, and loose fitting short-shorts for him can provide many moments of discreet summery pleasures.

TIPS
&
TRICKS

192

Both males and females can perform the "peaking" technique, which will strengthen and lengthen orgasms. As you sense you're at the edge of climax, stop moving until the intensity decreases. Then bring yourself back to the edge again, and pause again. Each time pause a little longer before bringing yourself to the brink. On the third go-round, go for it!

TIPS
&
TRICKS

193

A rule of thumb—or leg—for women: the higher you can lift your legs when you're underneath your man, the deeper his penetration will be. Use your legs to embrace him and pull him toward you with each stroke.

Tips
&
Tricks

For an excellent variation on the above, put your knees to your chest and drape your legs over his shoulders. Your vagina actually elongates when you do this, making room for the deeper thrusting to come.

Tips
&
Tricks

Many men's pleasure at orgasm will be enhanced when you lightly stroke from the small of the back up toward the shoulders and down again.

FACT:

Is it "her time of the month?" No, not *that* time— about a week before, in fact, she is in prime love-making mode. During the third week of a woman's cycle, when testosterone levels are at their peak, most women are, well, horny. Studies show they are more interested in lovemaking, more likely to masturbate, and will reach orgasm more easily.

Tips & Tricks

197

Here's an essential "FYI": this four-day span is also prime baby-making time. Isn't that just like Mother Nature? Be extra careful.

Tips & Tricks

198

Guys, try this orgasm booster. Right before ejaculating, have your partner press upward on your testicles *gently* with an open palm. This can heighten your arousal and add oomph to the Big Oh.

Tips & Tricks

199

Use gravity to enhance your climax by lying so that your head is lower than your heart. This can be done either by placing pillows under your hips or by letting your head hang slightly over the edge of the bed. These positions boost blood flow to the brain and change your breathing, which elevates arousal.

TIPS & TRICKS

200

Any time you are closely involved with his important parts (rubbing, licking, sucking, nuzzling), let him know how gorgeous he is and how much what you're doing turns you on.

TIPS & TRICKS

201

Acrobatics are not required for great sex. Although sexual experimentation can open new and exciting vistas for some, many couples enjoy satisfying long-term sexual relationships using only traditional methods.

202

Food For Thought

"It's been so long since I made love, I can't even remember who gets tied up."

—JOAN RIVERS, COMEDIENNE

203

FACT: The difference between naughty and kinky (or kinky and weird for that matter) is in the eyes of the participants. If neither of you is into extreme masochism or sadism, and neither is disturbed by your adventures, don't worry about it.

204

Food For Thought

"Conscience is the inner voice that warns us someone may be looking."

— H. L. MENCKEN, WRITER

205

TIPS & TRICKS Learn to be shameless—literally. The more you can relax and be yourself while making love to your partner, the better the sex will be.

206

FACT: The less distracted you are during sex, the better your chance of achieving the Big Oh.

Tips
&
Tricks

207

For best results, lock the door, take the phone off the hook, and focus, focus, focus.

IX

After the Oh...

As true connoisseurs of coitus know, those moments of closeness immediately following "the act" can be the sweetest. So don't be in a hurry to disturb the mood, you may be surprised at what develops...

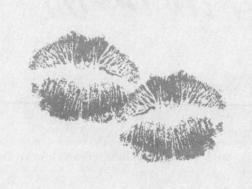

208

FACT: While it's true that men are more likely than women to become drowsy after sex, they are equally capable of enjoying post-coital closeness. These golden moments can be as satisfying in their own way as the fireworks that came first.

209

Food For Thought

"The only time human beings are sane is the ten minutes after intercourse."

— ERIC BERNE, PSYCHOLOGIST, AUTHOR OF *GAMES PEOPLE PLAY*

210

TIPS
&
TRICKS | Men are spent immediately after lovemaking and often their short and long term memory systems are down. So if he is responding, he's on automatic nod. Allow him his bliss, snuggle into his chest. He feels like a man now and any adoring actions on your part will enhance his feelings of well-being.

211

This is a good time for quiet, mutual pampering activity. In warm weather, have a basin of cool, scented water with two soft wash cloths nearby. Take turns wiping each other's brows and body parts. Remember, he's a guy; you can be firm and strong with your strokes, except those around his still-sensitive penis.

212

In the winter, do everything you can to stay cozy and snuggly after lovemaking. It's fun to crawl under a big down comforter and play survival on the tundra. You can make up the rules.

213

Men, try to remember that this is not the time to turn around and go to sleep. This is too rare and special a time to pass up in favor of napping. Talk a little, tell her what your favorite moments were. Tell her how you liked it when... Though this kind of talk may not come easily, the rewards in love, commitment—and more great sex—are profound.

214

As more time elapses, you might try to put his soft penis in your mouth and suck it gently and lovingly. He may not get hard again, but he'll most likely be quite receptive to any ideas you might have for continuing your pleasure time.

X

Nuptial Nookie

As most grown-ups know, "happily ever after" does not exactly capture the reality of relationships once a couple settles into the routine of marriage and family life. Couples who stay together past the euphoria of infatuation have found ways of sustaining—or at least periodically reawakening—those heady days of romance and passion.

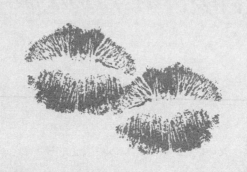

215

FACT: Monogamy is not instinctive in either sex (and is probably even less natural for men). However exciting it is in the beginning, sex with the same person can eventually become stale and predictable.

216

Food for Thought

"Of course platonic friendship is possible, but only between husband and wife."

—ATTRIBUTED TO POLITICAL WRITER, IRVING KRISTOL

217

TIPS
&
TRICKS

Make sex a priority. Sure, you're both busy; but unless you agree that your sex life is important and deserves your attention, the physical intimacy between you will fade away.

TIPS
&
TRICKS

218

Surprise your partner every now and then. Show up naked when he's reading or watching TV. He'll get the idea.

TIPS
&
TRICKS

219

Make love in a different room of the house. The bedroom may be the most comfortable, but the kitchen, dining room, foyer, or even the laundry room can make up in excitement what they lack in soft surfaces.

TIPS
&
TRICKS

220

If you and your partner are especially busy, make appointments for sex. When you set time aside, you ensure that sex doesn't get nudged completely off the list by soccer games, hair cuts, laundry, shopping, etc. Consider setting aside Friday evenings, Sunday afternoons, or any time you're usually together and have flexibility in your schedules.

221

You can surprise your mate in other ways, too. Wear a wig to your regularly scheduled sex appointment. You can pretend to be someone else, or act as if you're a complete stranger. Encourage your partner to join you in the spirit of fantasy and see what develops.

222

Vary your idea of what constitutes "sex." It doesn't always have to mean intercourse. Consider "quickies" with oral sex only, cuddling and touching sessions that may or may not lead to orgasm, or even make-out sessions that don't go beyond heavy petting.

223

Because sex is such an important part of the marital bond, find imaginative ways of reminding your beloved spouse how deeply you cherish that bond. Here's a verse from e.e. cummings that perfectly expresses this. You might want to write it out and tuck this poem in a place where you know your partner will find it.

> *i like my body when it is with your*
> *body. It is so quite new a thing.*
> *Muscles better and nerves more. . .*
> *And eyes big love-crumbs,*
> *and possibly i like the thrill*
> *of under me you so quite new*

224

Have each partner write secret sexual fantasies on separate index cards. Sort through the cards together and discuss each fantasy. Toss any that either partner finds uninteresting or distasteful. This experience can be an adventure in communication.

TIPS
&
TRICKS

225

Whenever you and your partner are feeling amorous, or adventuresome for that matter, pull out your stash of fantasy cards and try one.

TIPS
&
TRICKS

226

Don't limit your use of fantasy cards to the times when you're both feeling sexy. Those cards can work wonders when you're not feeling particularly lustful. Embarking on a fantasy session can really jumpstart sexual energy.

TIPS
&
TRICKS

227

If either of you is intimidated by suggesting sexual fantasies, or could use a little help with requests, turn to an erotic book for assistance. You can highlight appealing passages individually and review one another's notations together.

228

Food for Thought

*"If variety is the spice of life,
marriage is the big can of leftover Spam."*

— JOHNNY CARSON, TALK-SHOW HOST

229

TIPS
&
TRICKS

Give one another "sex checks"—coupons redeemable for special sexual encounters. You can make these yourself or order them from www.goodvibes.com.

230

TIPS
&
TRICKS

Use your racy imagination to come up with a variety of "Sex Check" ideas: "Naughty Night at the Movies" (X-rated videos at home), a promise of "Sex Anywhere, Anytime," or anything else you know will be a turn-on for you and your partner.

231

FACT: Abstinence can awaken a drowsy libido. Even if sex
has been so low on your priority list that you think
avoiding it for a week will be easy, you may be in for
a surprise.

TIPS
&
TRICKS

232

Abstain from sex for a week or so to build sexual
tension. While you're awaiting that red-letter day,
do your wicked best to arouse lust in one another.

TIPS
&
TRICKS

233

Exchange massages, share double-bubble baths, wear
sexy lingerie (or no underwear at all), indulge in
steamy, lingering kisses—but nothing more! This is
one occasion when frustrating your partner is the
actual goal!

234

Challenge your mate to an arousing game of competitive deep kissing (who can last longer without begging for more).

235

Food For Thought

"I've only slept with the men I've been married to. How many women can make that claim?"

—ELIZABETH TAYLOR (HILTON WILDING TODD FISHER BURTON WARNER FORTENSKY)

236

FACT: Studies of sexual relationships between long-time committed partners have shown that the higher the level of trust, the more satisfying the sex. By the same token, lovemaking can evaporate when anger or hurt feelings lurk just beneath the surface.

237

Be sure to talk with your partner about your sexual relationship from time to time. You may not be bored right now, but your lover could be. And how will you know unless you ask?

238

Food for Thought

"Assumptions are the termites of relationships."

— HENRY WINKLER, ACTOR

239

Make honest communication a habit— whether you're discussing sex or the check book. Stick to statements that describe your own feelings when talking to your partner and avoid using words like "always" and "never."

240

Tips & Tricks

If you are the person initiating change in your love-making routine and your partner has some doubts, be gradual in your approach. Incremental change is less threatening than radical departure from long-established habit.

241

Tips & Tricks

Keep sex high enough on the radar screen so that you are regularly talking about it, doing it, or fooling around in a way that may or may not lead up to it.

242

Tips & Tricks

In addition to being the most fun you can have without laughing (as Woody Allen says in *Annie Hall*), sex is also a sublime method of communication between lovers and can lead to deepening intimacy. Under ideal circumstances—which may or may not include lingerie, sex toys, candles, bubble baths, etc. —the rewards of good sex extend well beyond the thrill of the moment.